Copyright 2023

All right reserved. No part of this book should be resproduce without express permission of the author.

Reproduction of all or any part of this book is punishable under relevant law.

Table of Contents

PREVIEW
The word carnivore is derived from Latin and literally means
"meat eater."

A carnivore is an animal that feeds on other animals.

Carnivores come in many shapes in sizes, but they often have
some similarities. Most carnivores have relatively large
brains and high levels of intelligence. They also have less
complicated digestive systems than herbivores. The world's
largest animal is also the world's largest carnivore.

A mammal that eats only the meat from other animals is a
carnivore. In the wild, a carnivore will hunt other animals for
food. Carnivores usually have to eat a lot to give them the
energy they need. Sometimes these animals have to spend
most of their days hunting to make sure they get enough
food. Because carnivores need to cut and tear up their food,
they have big canine teeth and sharp molars. Carnivores
usually have small incisors in the front of their mouths. Big
carnivores include lions, tigers, and wolves. Some birds such
as hawks and eagles are also carnivores. Snakes are usually
carnivores as well. Small carnivores include frogs, birds such
as robins, and spiders. Carnivores provide an important
service in the wild because they help control the population
of other animals. If carnivores were not hunting and
removing these animals from environments, these animals
could overpopulate an area.

BREAKFAST
1. Keto Breakfast Sandwich with Pancakes

Prep Time: 10 Minutes

Cook Time: 20 Minutes

Servings: 2

Ingredients

- ½ lb ground breakfast sausage
- Pancakes
- 2 tablespoon Coconut flour or ¼ cup almond flour
- 2 large eggs
- 1 teaspoon baking powder
- 1 ½ tablespoon oil
- 1 tablespoon sugar free maple syrup
- pinch of salt
- cooking spray
- eggs
- 4 large eggs
- 1 tablespoon butter
- kosher salt to taste
- garnish
- sugar free maple syrup
- butter

Instructions

1. Patty up the breakfast sausage into 2 patties and place in a cast iron skillet over medium high heat. Cook on

each side until a crust forms and an internal
temperature reads 145F

2. Low Carb Hash

Prep Time: 20 Minutes

Cook Time: 20 Minutes

Servings: 4

Ingredients

- 7 Slices Thick Bacon , Cut in Lardons
- 4 Cups Celeriac , Diced
- 1 Orange Bell Pepper , Diced
- 1 Zucchini , Diced
- ½ teaspoon Onion Powder
- ½ teaspoon Smoked Paprika
- ¼ teaspoon Oregano
- Kosher salt and pepper to taste
- 4 Large Eggs
- Avocado and Parsley for Garnish

Instructions

2. Saute bacon lardons in a cast iron or heavy bottom skillet over medium heat until crisp. Remove from the pan leaving grease
3. Add celeriac to the pan and sauté for 5 minutes
4. Add orange pepper and sauté for 5 minutes more
5. Add zucchini, onion powder, paprika, oregano, and salt and pepper and sauté until zucchini is cooked through
6. Crack each egg on top of the veggies leaving the yolk intact

7. Cover skillet with lid and continue to cook until egg whites are set. About 5 minutes
8. Garnish with chopped parsley and diced avocado
9. Servings: 4 servings

3. Low Carb Casserole

Prep Time: 5 Minutes

Cook Time: 35 Minutes

Servings: 6

Ingredients

- 12 large Eggs, Beaten
- ½ Cup Half and Half
- ½ teaspoon Kosher salt
- ¼ teaspoon Pepper
- 2 cups Shredded cheddar cheese
- 1 tablespoon avocado oil
- 3 cloves Garlic, minced
- 8 ounces Mushrooms, sliced
- 5 ounces Raw baby spinach
- 4 Slices Thick cut bacon, cooked and cut into 2 inch pieces

Instructions

1. Pre-heat the oven to 375F and spray a 9 x 9 casserole with cooking spray
2. In a large mixing bowl, add the eggs, half and half, salt, and pepper. Whisk thoroughly. Add in the cheese
3. In a large skillet over medium heat, add oil and garlic. Sauté for 1 minute. Add in the mushrooms and sauté for 1 minute more. Finally, add in the spinach and mix in with the mushrooms. Continue to sauté until the spinach is wilted. Remove from the heat.

4. Add the spinach and mushrooms to the bowl with the eggs. Mix to combine. Pour into the greased casserole and lay the bacon pieces on top.
5. Bake in the pre-heated oven for 30 minutes or until the casserole is set in the middle.
6. Serve hot, or wrap portions in foil or plastic wrap and store in the fridge up to 1 week.
7. Jennifer's tips
8. You can easily double this recipe and use a 9 x 13 casserole dish. Bake for 45 minutes or until set.
9. You can definitely use heavy cream instead of half and half if you want a lower carb count.
10. You can add cooked sausage or crumbled bacon into the casserole. I would use ½ pound of sausage cooked and crumbled, or 6 slices of bacon cooked and crumbled. Add it to the egg mixture with the mushrooms and spinach.
11. To check the low carb breakfast casserole for doneness...insert a butter knife into the middle of the casserole and check to see if the egg is set.
12. This keto breakfast casserole is perfect for freezing. You can bake the casserole in a foil pan, let cool, cover with foil and then freeze, or you can bake it, let cool, remove it from the pan, wrap very well in foil, and freeze.

Prep Time: 10 Minutes

Cook Time: 40 Minutes

Servings: 10

Ingredients

- 8 Ounces keto bread (I use Sola), cubed
- 12 Large eggs
- 2 Cups half and half
- 1 teaspoon Kosher salt
- ½ teaspoon pepper
- 16 Ounces ground breakfast sausage, cooked and crumbled
- 1 ½ Cups Shredded sharp cheddar cheese
- ½ Cup Shredded Parmesan Cheese
- 1 Cup sliced mushrooms

Instructions

1. Preheat the oven to 400F and spray a 9x13 casserole dish with cooking spray. Take a baking sheet and spread out the bread cubes. Place into the oven and bake for about 8 minutes, or until toasted. Set the bread aside to cool. Lower the oven to 350F.
2. In a large mixing bowl, whisk together the eggs, half and half, salt, and pepper. Stir in the cooked sausage, both cheeses, and the toasted bread.
3. Pour the mixture into the casserole dish, top with the sliced mushrooms, and bake in the oven for 40-50 minutes or until the center is completely set.

5. Low Carb Burrito for One

Prep Time: 5 Minutes

Cook Time: 10 Minutes

Servings: 1

Ingredients

- 1 Low Carb tortilla (I use La Banderita carb counter soft taco size)
- 1 large egg
- 1 guacamole cup (I use a Wholly guacamole mini cup)
- 2 pre-cooked breakfast sausage links (I use Jones Chicken Sausages)
- ¼ cup shredded cheddar cheese
- 2 tablespoons taco sauce (for dipping)

Instructions

1. Crack the egg in a medium non-stick skillet over medium heat and scramble it with a small silicone spatula until cooked through, about 5 minutes. Heat the sausage according to the package directions.
2. Lay out the tortilla on a large plate and layer your cheese over half the tortilla, followed by the cooked egg, guacamole, and sausage. Fold in the sides and roll into a burrito.
3. Using the same skillet you used for the egg, turn to medium heat and heat the burrito seam side down until it is lightly browned. Flip and repeat for the other side. Serve with taco sauce.
4. Jennifer's tips

5. If you do not have Wholly Guacamole, you can use 2 ounces of smashed avocado
6. If you are on the go, you can put your taco sauce inside the burrito.
7. For on the go, you can wrap this in foil or plastic wrap.

6. Shirred Eggs with Prosciutto and Parmesan

Prep Time: 5 Minutes

Cook Time: 12 Minutes

Servings: 1

Ingredients

- 1 Tablespoon heavy whipping cream
- 2 large eggs
- Kosher salt and pepper to taste
- 1 Slice Prosciutto
- 1 Tablespoon grated parmesan cheese

Instructions

1. Preheat the oven to 375F and spray the inside of an 8 ounce ramekin with cooking spray. Pour the whipping cream into ramekin.
2. Crack each egg into the ramekin. Nestle the prosciutto around the eggs. Season with salt and pepper and then top with parmesan cheese.
3. Place ramekin into the oven and bake until the egg white is set. Should take about 12-15 minutes. For firm yolks bake for an additional 3 minutes. Let sit for a few minutes to set and serve. Enjoy!

Prep Time: 5 Minutes

Cook Time: 10 Minutes

Servings: 2

Ingredients

- 2 Eggs
- 2 scoops Whey Protein powder
- 1 teaspoon Baking powder
- 6 Tablespoons Water or Almond milk
- Cooking spray, butter, or coconut oil for greasing the pan

Instructions

1. Place a non-stick skillet on the stove over medium heat. Spray with cooking spray or use butter or coconut oil and let melt.
2. Mix the eggs, protein powder, and baking powder in a large bowl. Add the water or almond milk a little at a time until the batter is pancake batter consistency. You may not need all of the water.
3. Using a ⅓ cup measure, pour out the batter into the skillet. I was able to make 3 at a time. They are ready to flip when bubble start to form on the top.
4. Serve with butter, sugar free syrup, and chocolate chips.
5. Jennifer's tips
6. The nutrition listed is for the Premiere Vanilla Protein powder

7. You can try this with other protein powders but I cannot guarantee it will work. I have heard that Quest protein powder also works well for protein recipes. It really needs to be a protein powder that tastes good on it's own!

Prep Time: 10 Minutes

Cook Time: 20 Minutes

Servings: 4

Ingredients

- 1 cup almond flour
- 1 tablespoon Granular Sweetener
- 1 teaspoon baking powder
- 2 large eggs, separated
- ½ cup unsweetened almond milk
- 1 teaspoon vanilla

Instructions

1. In a large mixing bowl, stir together the almond flour, sweetener, and baking powder until well combined. Stir in 1 egg yolk, the almond milk, and vanilla. (Reserve the other egg yolk for another purpose) Set aside the batter.
2. In a small mixing bowl, beat the egg whites using a hand mixer until stiff peaks form. Fold the whites into the pancake batter. Let the pancake batter sit for 5 minutes to thicken.
3. Grease a nonstick griddle or large nonstick skillet with cooking spray or oil and heat over medium heat. Pour ¼ cup portions of the batter into the skillet or on the griddle and let cook until bubbles start to form on the edges, about 3 minutes, then carefully flip and continue cooking until slightly golden, about 2

minutes. Repeat with the remaining batter. Serve with your favorite keto toppings (I like butter and sugar-free syrup).

Prep Time: 2 Minutes

Cook Time: 5 Minutes

Servings: 1

Ingredients

- ½ Cup Protein powder
- 1 Egg
- 3 Tablespoons Plain fat free Greek Yogurt or sour cream
- 1 teaspoon Baking powder
- pinch of salt
- butter and sugar free syrup for serving

Instructions

1. Heat your waffle iron on medium and spray with cooking spray.
2. Mix the protein powder, egg, Greek Yogurt, baking powder, and salt in a medium sized bowl until fully combined.
3. Pour half of the batter in the waffle iron (for smaller waffle irons, pour less batter), and cook according to your waffle irons directions.
4. Serve with butter and sugar free syrup.
5. Jennifer's tips
6. Nutritional information is calculated using the vanilla protein powder and plain fat free Greek Yogurt.

7. You can try this with other protein powders but I cannot guarantee it will work. I have heard that Quest protein powder works well for protein recipes.
8. I updated this recipe to using sour cream instead of water. I found the resulting waffles to be even tastier.

Prep Time: 5 Minutes

Cook Time: 20 Minutes

Servings: 12

Ingredients

- 2 ½ Cups almond flour
- 1 teaspoon Baking soda
- ¼ teaspoon Kosher salt
- ½ Cup Granular Sweetener
- 3 Large Eggs, beaten
- 8 ounces Unsweetened Greek Yogurt
- 2 teaspoons Vanilla Extract
- 1 Cup Blueberries

Instructions

1. Preheat your oven to 400F and line a 12 cup muffin pan with liners. Make sure you spray the inside of the liners with cooking spray.
2. In a large mixing bowl, combine your almond flour, baking soda, salt and sweetener. Now you can add the beaten eggs, greek yogurt and vanilla extract. Lastly, fold in your blueberries.
3. Scoop your batter into the muffin cups evenly using a scoop or spoon. Bake in the oven for 15-18 minutes or until a toothpick comes out clean.
4. Jennifer's tips
5. Allergic to almonds: Try sunflower seed flour or peanut flour

6. What can you use instead of Greek Yogurt: Sour cream is a perfect replacement
7. Can you use frozen blueberries: Yes, they will work perfectly

11. Keto "Oatmeal" Cookies - 2 Net Carbs!

Prep Time: 10 Minutes

Cook Time: 12 Minutes

Servings: 12

Ingredients

- 1 ½ cups almond flour
- 2 Tablespoons Coconut flour
- ½ Cup Granular Sweetener
- 1 teaspoon Baking powder
- 1 teaspoon ground cinnamon
- ½ teaspoon Kosher salt
- ½ Cup Melted Butter
- 2 Large Eggs
- 1 teaspoon Vanilla
- ½ Cup Sliced almonds
- ½ Cup Hemp hearts

Instructions

1. Pre-heat the oven to 350F. Line a sheet pan with parchment or a silicone baking mat. You may need 2 cookie sheets.
2. Combine the dry ingredients: almond flour, sweetener, coconut flour, baking powder, cinnamon, and salt in a large mixing bowl. Now stir in the wet ingredients. Finally, stir in the almonds or hemp hearts (or oats if using)

3. Scoop out the mix into 16 even sized cookies and place on the sheet pan 2 inches apart. Flatten the tops with your fingers. Bake in the oven for 12-13 minutes, or until the bottom edges start to turn golden brown.
4. Remove from the oven and let cool completely. Store on the counter in an airtight container for up to 3 days, or in the refrigerator for up to 1 week.
5. Jennifer's tips
6. Freezing: After the keto oatmeal cookies are finished baking, leave them on the sheet pan and put them in the freezer for 1 hour to flash freeze, then put them in freezer safe airtight container and store in the freezer for up to 3 months.
7. let's say you did want to use 1 cup of oats instead of the almonds and hemp hearts. That would reduce the calories to 148 per cookie and the carbs would go from 4 grams to 6 bringing the net carbs to 4 grams.
8. This recipe is my original keto breakfast cookies recipe. The only difference is the addition of the cinnamon.

Prep Time: 10 Minutes

Cook Time: 20 Minutes

Servings: 6

Ingredients

- ½ pound ground breakfast sausage
- 8 Eggs, beaten
- ½ cup Diced green bell pepper
- ½ cup Diced white onion
- ½ cup Shredded Parmesan Cheese
- 2 tablespoons Chopped parsley
- ½ cup Heavy cream

Instructions

1. Preheat oven to 425F.
2. Heat a 10 inch oven proof skillet over medium heat. I use cast iron.
3. Add in sausage, onion and bell pepper.
4. Cook and crumble sausage until sausage is cooked through and onion and bell peppr are soft. 5-8 minutes
5. In a large bowl, mix together eggs, parmesan cheese, heavy cream and parsley.
6. Pour egg mixtue on top of sausage mixture and stir. Let cook for 2-3 minutes.
7. Remove skillet from heat and place skillet in preheated oven for 20 to 30 minutes or until the center of the frittata is set.

8. Cut into 6 servings and serve.

Prep Time: 10 Minutes

Cook Time: 10 Minutes

Servings: 4

Ingredients

Salad:

- 6 Cups Shredded Tri-color Chopped Cabbage slaw mix
- 1 Medium red bell pepper, cut into thin strips
- 3 green onions, sliced
- ¼ Cup Chopped fresh cilantro
- ½ cup peanuts, chopped

Sesame Ginger Dressing:

- 4 Tablespoon sesame oil
- 2 Tablespoon Rice vinegar
- 2 Tablespoon Keto honey substitute
- 2 Tablespoon lime juice
- 2 teaspoon ginger paste
- 1 teaspoon kosher salt
- ½ teaspoon Ground black pepper

Instructions

1. Combine all of the salad ingredients in a large mixing bowl.

2. In a medium size mixing bowl, whisk together all of
    the dressing ingredients. Pour over the salad
    ingredients and toss to combine.

14. Shirred Eggs with Prosciutto and Parmesan

Prep Time: 5 Minutes

Cook Time: 12 Minutes

Servings: 1

Ingredients

- 1 Tablespoon heavy whipping cream
- 2 large eggs
- Kosher salt and pepper to taste
- 1 Slice Prosciutto
- 1 Tablespoon grated parmesan cheese

Instructions

1. Preheat the oven to 375F and spray the inside of an 8 ounce ramekin with cooking spray. Pour the whipping cream into ramekin.
2. Crack each egg into the ramekin. Nestle the prosciutto around the eggs. Season with salt and pepper and then top with parmesan cheese.
3. Place ramekin into the oven and bake until the egg white is set. Should take about 12-15 minutes. For firm yolks bake for an additional 3 minutes. Let sit for a few minutes to set and serve. Enjoy!

15. Tex-Mex Chicken and Veggies

Prep Time: 10 Minutes

Cook Time: 20 Minutes

Servings: 6

Ingredients

- 1 Tablespoon avocado oil
- 1 medium onion, diced
- 3 Garlic cloves, minced
- 1 Medium Bell Pepper, diced
- 2 Pounds boneless skinless thighs- cut into 1" pieces
- 2 medium Zucchini, diced
- 14 Ounce can Fire roasted diced tomatoes
- ¼ Cup chopped cilantro
- 1 ½ Tablespoons Taco Seasoning
- 1 ½ Cups Colby Jack Cheese, divided for serving

Instructions

1. Heat the avocado oil in a large skillet over medium-high heat. stir in the onion, garlic and bell pepper. Sauté for 5 minutes or until the onion is translucent.
2. Move the veggies to one side of your skillet and add in the chicken. Cook for about 5 minutes, stirring occasionally.
3. Next add your fire roasted tomatoes, zucchini, cilantro and taco seasoning. Stir and cook on medium-low for 10 minutes or until the veggies are tender.
4. Serve topped with cheese. Makes 6 servings

16. Garlic Butter Shrimp with Cauliflower Rice

Prep Time: 10 Minutes

Cook Time: 20 Minutes

Servings: 6

Ingredients

- 1 ½ lbs Raw large frozen shrimp thawed, peeled, and deveined
- 20 ounces Riced cauliflower
- ½ cup Salted butter, melted
- 1 tablespoon minced garlic
- 2 teaspoon dried, chopped, parsley
- ½ teaspoon Kosher salt
- ¼ teaspoon fresh ground black pepper

Instructions

1. Pre-heat oven to 400F
2. Cut the florets off of the stem of the cauliflower and discard the stem. Add the florets to a food processor and process until it resembles the texture of rice. Alternatively, you can buy already riced cauliflower in the fresh or frozen section of the supermarket. If your "rice" is frozen and in chunks, place in a microwave safe container and microwave in 30 second intervals until the chunks can break apart.
3. In a large bowl, add thawed and cleaned shrimp, butter, garlic, parsley, salt and black pepper. Mix to combine

4. Add the riced cauliflower to the bowl and mix to combine.
5. Pour the shrimp and cauliflower mixture onto a sheet pan, making sure the shrimp are in a single layer. Bake in the oven for 15 minutes. Makes 4 servings

Prep Time: 10 Minutes

Cook Time: 1hr 10 Minutes

Servings: 4

Ingredients

- 3 Tablespoons unsalted butter
- 2 yellow onion, peeled and thinly sliced
- ½ teaspoon kosher salt
- 4 cups beef broth
- ½ cup pumpkin puree
- ½ teaspoon black pepper
- 4 slices your favorite bread (I use Sola bread for low carb) each cut in a circle
- 4 slices Swiss cheese, chopped

Instructions

1. Melt the butter in a medium sized dutch oven over medium heat. Stir in the onions and ½ teaspoon kosher salt and cover with a lid. Let the onions cook for about 5 minutes to start to soften. Remove the lid and let the onions caramelize until golden brown, stirring occasionally. This will take 45-60 minutes.
2. Once onions are caramelized, stir in the broth and pumpkin puree. Season with pepper and salt to taste. Bring to a boil for about 10 minutes.
3. Set your broiler to high and arrange individual 8 ounce ramekins on a baking sheet. Using a ladle, spoon onion soup into ramekins evenly and cover top

with bread slices. Place one slice of swiss cheese over each ramekin. Broil for a minute or two or until cheese is melted and browned. Serve.

Prep Time: 10 Minutes

Cook Time: 20 Minutes

Servings: 12

Ingredients

- 2 ½ Cups almond flour
- ½ Cup Granular Sweetener
- 1 teaspoon Baking soda
- 1 teaspoon pumpkin pie spice
- ¼ teaspoon kosher salt
- 3 Large Eggs, beaten
- ½ cup fat free plain Greek yogurt
- ½ Cup pumpkin puree
- 2 teaspoons Vanilla Extract

Instructions

1. Preheat the oven to 400F and line a 12 cup muffin pan with liners. Spray the inside of your liners with cooking spray. Set aside.
2. In a large mixing bowl, combine the almond flour, baking soda, salt, pumpkin pie spice and sweetener. Next add in your beaten eggs, greek yogurt, vanilla extract and pumpkin purée. Mix until all your ingredients are combined.
3. Using a scoop or spoon, evenly distribute your pumpkin muffin batter into each muffin cup. Place into already preheated oven and bake for 15-20

minutes or until a toothpick comes out clean. Serve
and enjoy!

Prep Time: 10 Minutes

Cook Time: 20 Minutes

Servings: 10

Ingredients

- 1 Pound Ground pork sausage
- 2 Cups Shredded Cheddar Cheese
- 1.5 Cups almond flour
- 2 teaspoons Dried parsley
- 1 teaspoon Smoked paprika
- 2 teaspoons Baking powder

Instructions

1. Pre-heat the oven to 350F. Prepare a large baking sheet by covering with a silicone baking mat or parchment paper.
2. Combine all ingredients in a large bowl and mix thoroughly. Using a 1 tablespoon cookie scoop, portion out the mixture and roll into balls. Place on the baking sheet about 1 inch apart. Makes about 40 balls
3. Bake in the preheated oven for 20 minutes or until the internal temperature reaches 145F
4. Jennifer's tips
5. Cover your rimmed baking tray with a silicone mat or parchment paper for easy cleanup.
6. Use a 2 tablespoon scoop for easy and even portioning of the keto sausage balls.

7. Use sharp cheddar cheese for a nice sharp bite.

20. Chicken, Mushrooms, and Cauliflower Rice

Prep Time: 10 Minutes

Cook Time: 15 Minutes

Servings: 4

Ingredients

- 2 Tablespoons avocado oil
- 2 stalks Celery, diced
- ½ cup Shredded carrots
- 8 ounces Baby Bella mushrooms, sliced
- ½ teaspoon kosher salt
- ¼ teaspoon Dried Thyme
- 1 ½ Pounds Chicken Breast, cut into 1 inch chunks
- 10 Ounces frozen cauliflower rice
- salt and pepper

Instructions

1. Heat the avocado oil in a large skillet over medium heat. Stir in the diced celery and shredded carrots. Cook for 5-8 minutes or until translucent.
2. Stir in the sliced mushrooms, salt, and dried thyme. Cook for about 5 minutes.
3. Stir in the chicken breast chunks and cook for about 8 minutes. Stir in your cauliflower rice, stirring to mix all your ingredients. Once cooked through, season with salt and pepper to taste. Enjoy!
4. Jennifer's tips
5. Meal prep this recipe

6. This recipe is so simple to meal prep! I like to divide
    it evenly into 4 meal prep containers and then I have
    lunch or dinner for 4 days. You could even freeze this
    recipe for up to a few months in freezer safe
    containers.

21. Sheet Pan Chicken Sausage and Peppers

Prep Time: 10 Minutes

Cook Time: 20 Minutes

Servings: 4

Ingredients

- 1 Yellow bell pepper, cut into strips
- 1 Orange bell pepper, sliced
- 1 Large Sweet Onion, sliced
- 2 Tablespoons avocado oil
- ½ tablespoon Italian seasoning
- 1 teaspoon garlic powder
- 1 teaspoon kosher salt
- ½ teaspoon freshly ground black pepper
- 4 Chicken Sausage Links I use Aidells

Instructions

1. Preheat oven to 400F and line a sheet pan with parchment paper or aluminum foil. Add the chopped peppers and onions to the pan and drizzle with the oil. Sprinkle the seasonings over top and then use tongs to toss the oil and seasonings with the peppers and onions. Spread the mixture evenly around the sheet pan and finally, arrange the sausages on top.
2. Place into already preheated oven and bake for 20-25 minutes, until the sausages are browned and the onions and peppers are wilted and starting to brown

around the edges. Serve with your favorite hot dog buns...I like Lewis Bake shop for low carb

22. Keto Sesame Chicken

Prep Time: 5 Minutes

Cook Time: 11 Minutes

Servings: 4

Ingredients

- 1.5 pounds boneless skinless chicken breasts, cut into 1 inch pieces
- 5 Tablespoons Soy sauce
- ¼ Cup Ketchup (sugar free for keto)
- 2 cloves garlic, minced
- ¼ Cup Brown Sugar Sweetener
- ½ teaspoon onion powder
- 1 Tablespoon sesame oil
- ¼ teaspoon red pepper flakes
- sesame seeds for garnish

Instructions

1. In a small mixing bowl, combine the soy sauce, ketchup, minced garlic, brown sugar, onion powder, sesame oil and red pepper flakes. Stir to combine ingredients and set aside.
2. Heat a non stick skillet over medium high heat. Add your chicken breast chunks. Cook until slightly brown and cooked through, should take about 5-8 minutes. Test the internal temperature with a meat probe thermometer to make sure the chicken is 165F.
3. Pour the sauce over the chicken and stir to coat. Turn your heat down to medium low and let simmer for

about 5 minutes to thicken. Serve topped with sesame seeds for garnish.

4. Jennifer's tips
5. Make this a freezer meal: To make this keto sesame chicken a freezer meal, simply place the chopped raw chicken in a freezer safe zip top bag along with the combined sauce ingredients. store flat in the freezer for up to 4 months. When you are ready to cook, remove from the freezer the night before and let thaw in the refrigerator. Pour the contents of the bag into a skillet over medium heat and stir until the chicken is cooked through.

23. Steak Chili - Low Carb Chili

Prep Time: 10 Minutes

Cook Time: 20 Minutes

Servings: 6

Ingredients

- 1 Tablespoons avocado oil
- 1 ½ Pounds Sirloin Steak, cut into 1 inch cubes
- kosher salt and black pepper to taste
- ½ Onion, diced
- 6 Cloves Garlic, minced
- 2 Tablespoons tomato paste
- 1 Cup beef broth
- 2 Tablespoons chili powder
- 1 Tablespoon garlic powder
- 1 Tablespoon Cumin
- 2 Tablespoons smoked paprika
- 28 Ounces Canned fire roasted crushed tomatoes
- 15 Ounces Canned black Soy Beans, drained and rinsed (or bean of choice)

Instructions

1. Heat the oil in a large heavy bottom pot over medium-high heat. Stir in steak, season with salt and pepper, and cook steak until browned on all sides, about 5 minutes. Remove from the pot to a plate and set aside.
2. Reduce the heat to medium and stir in the chopped onion and garlic. Sauté until translucent, about 5 minutes. Stir in the tomato paste, beef broth, and

spices. Scrape any browned bits from the bottom of the pan and cook the spices for a few minutes.

3. Stir in the already cooked steak, crushed tomatoes, and beans. Let simmer for 5 minutes. Season with salt and black pepper to taste. Garnish with cheddar cheese and sour cream if desired.

4. Jennifer's tips

5. Be sure to cut your steak into bite sized pieces for easier eating. No one wants to have to eat low carb chili with a fork and knife!

6. Use a large dutch oven so you can brown all of the meat in one or two batches. I like my large oval dutch oven for this.

7. Smoked paprika really gives an amazing flavor to this low carb steak chili. You can usually find it in most large grocery stores.

8. Add some cayenne pepper or diced jalapeño peppers for an extra kick.

9. Store: Keep the steak chili in an airtight container in the refrigerator for up to 1 week.

10. Freeze: The low carb chili can be frozen in a freezer safe zip top bag or freezer safe airtight container for up to 3 months.

11. Meal prep: Divide the steak chili evenly between 6 meal prep containers with tight fitting lids. Store in the refrigerator for up to 1 week. Microwave according to the meal prep containers instructions.

Prep Time: 20 Minutes

Cook Time: 00 Minutes

Servings: 4

Ingredients

Italian Dressing:

- ⅓ Cup olive oil
- 3 Tablespoons red wine vinegar
- 1 teasooon Granular Sweetener
- 1 Clove garlic, minced
- 1 teaspoon Dijon Mustard
- 1 teaspoon italian seasoning
- ½ teaspoon kosher salt
- pepper to taste

Salad:

- 12 cups Chopped Romaine Lettuce
- 6 Ounces Genoa Salami, cut into 4ths
- 1 ½ Cup cherry tomatoes, cut in half
- ½ Cup sliced black olives
- ¼ Cup sliced pepperoncinis
- ½ Cup chopped provolone cheese
- ¼ Cup shredded parmesan
- ½ small red onion, thinly sliced

Instructions

1. To make the Italian Dressing, combine in a small mixing bowl, olive oil, red wine vinegar, sweetener, garlic, dijon, italian seasoning, salt and pepper. Whisk together to combine all your ingredients. Set aside.
2. In a large salad bowl, start building your salad by adding in your chopped romaine lettuce, salami, cherry tomatoes, sliced olives, sliced pepperoncinis, sliced onions, provolone cheese and shredded parmesan.
3. Using salad tongs, toss your salad to combine all your ingredients. Add your homemade italian dressing and toss to coat. Serve and enjoy!
4. Jennifer's tips
5. Store: If you know the whole salad isn't going to be consumed in one sitting, do not toss the salad with dressing. Store the romaine, toppings, and dressing all separately for the best results.
6. Meal prep: To meal prep this keto salad, separate the chopped romaine into a meal prep bowl. You can put the toppings on top of the lettuce, or you can separate them into their own bowl or zip top bag. The dressing can be stored in a small portable dressing cup. This salad meal prep container makes a meal prep salad a breeze!

Prep Time: 5 Minutes

Cook Time: 25 Minutes

Servings: 6

Ingredients

- 1 medium spaghetti squash yield 3 cups of noodles
- 1 tablespoon avocado oil
- 1 cup diced celery
- 1 cup shredded carrots
- 6 boneless skinless chicken thighs, chopped into 1 inch pieces
- ½ teaspoon Kosher salt
- ½ teaspoon fresh cracked black pepper
- ½ teaspoon dried basil
- ½ teaspoon dried thyme
- ¼ cup soy sauce (or Tamari for gluten free)
- 8 cups chicken broth
- 3 scallions (green parts only) sliced

Instructions

1. Pre-heat the oven to 425F and line a large baking tray with foil or parchment paper. Using a sharp knife, poke 1 to 2 holes in the spaghetti squash and place on a microwave safe plate. Microwave for 5 minutes. Let cool enough to handle.
2. Using a sharp knife, cut the squash into 1 inch rings and place on the baking pan in a single layer. Roast for 20-25 minutes until tender. When finished

cooking, scrape and discard the seeds from the center of the spaghetti squash rings, then shred the squash noodles from the skin.

3. While the squash is cooking, make the soup. Add the oil to a large heavy bottom pot over medium heat. Add the celery and carrots and sauté until soft. About 5 minutes. Add the chicken, season with salt and pepper, and cook for 8 minutes, stirring occasionally.

4. Season with basil and thyme and stir in the soy sauce. Use a wooden spoon to scrape any browned bits from the bottom of the pan. Now stir in the chicken broth and let simmer for a few minutes. Finally, stir in the spaghetti squash noodles.

5. Serve with sliced scallions.

6. Jennifer's tips

7. Use a whole chicken: For a truly healing keto chicken soup, instead of boneless skinless chicken thighs, you can use a whole chicken to make your own broth. Simply simmer a whole chicken in 8 cups of water for at least 1 hour. Make sure to season with salt to taste. Strain the broth and pull the chicken from the bones. Discard the bones and skin, or save for chicken bone broth.

8. Use a rotisserie chicken: For an even easier keto chicken soup, pull the chicken from a rotisserie chicken and use that in place of the chicken thighs.

9. Different vegetable noodles: Use zucchini noodles in place of spaghetti squash noodles like in this Chicken Meatball and Zoodle Soup.

Prep Time: 10 Minutes

Cook Time: 20 Minutes

Servings: 1

Ingredients

- 4 ounces cooked chicken breast, chopped
- ¼ Cup Buffalo Sauce
- 2 Cups chopped romaine
- ⅓ Cup halved cherry tomatoes
- ¼ Cup crumbled bleu cheese
- 1 small piece of red onion, thinly sliced
- 2 tablespoons chopped celery
- ¼ Cup shredded carrot
- ¼ Avocado, sliced
- 2 tablespoons Greek Yogurt Ranch or your favorite ranch dressing

Instructions

1. In a medium mixing bowl, combine the already cooked chicken and buffalo sauce. Toss to coat chicken. Set aside.
2. In a salad bowl or large plate, begin building your salad. Add in your already chopped romaine lettuce, shredded carrot, cherry tomatoes, crumbled bleu cheese and thinly sliced onion. Next add your chicken tossed in buffalo sauce, top with greek yogurt ranch dressing. Serve and enjoy!
3. Jennifer's tips

4. Nutrition does not include dressing
5. When it comes to meal prepping salads, especially this buffalo chicken salad, you need to remember just a few things.
6. Keep all of your wet ingredients operate from your dry ingredients. This chicken in this recipe is wet from the buffalo sauce. I would keep that in a separate container. I would also keep the blue cheese in a separate container because it can potentially make your lettuce soggy.
7. Keep your dressings in a separate container from your vegetables so everything stays fresh. All of the vegetables can be stored together.

Prep Time: 5 Minutes

Cook Time: 55 Minutes

Servings: 4

Ingredients

- 1 Large Spaghetti Squash
- 8 ounces feta cheese block
- 20 ounces cherry tomatoes
- 2 tablespoons avocado oil
- 2 tablespoons chopped fresh basil leaves
- ½ teaspoon kosher salt and pepper

Instructions

Spaghetti Squash Noodles

1. Preheat the oven to 400F. To make the squash easier to cut, poke a large hole in it with a knife and microwave for 5 minutes. Cut your squash in half lengthwise, remove the seeds with a spoon, and season with salt. Place on a baking sheet and roast for 20-40 minutes or until tender. Test for tenderness by poking a fork throught the flesh. It should penetrate easily. Set aside.
2. Place the feta cheese in the middle of a 9x13 casserole dosh. Place your cheery tomatoes around feta, and sprinkle the chopped basil on top. Drizzle the avocado oil over the top and season with salt and pepper.

3. Bake for 30 minutes or until tomatoes burst. Take out of oven and use a fork to carefully smash the tomatoes and mix with the baked feta.
4. Use a fork to shred the spaghetti squash in the shells. Top with the baked feta and tomato mixture.
5. Jennifer's tips
6. Nutrition information is for 1 cup of cooked spaghetti squash and ¼th of the sauce.
7. Grape tomatoes would work in this recipe if you cannot find cherry tomatoes.
8. The brick feta is packed in water so you will want to drain off the water. I suppose this would work just as well with crumbled feta but I haven't tried it. I don't see why not though!
9. Fresh basil really elevates the flavor of this dish so I wouldn't skip it.

28. Thai Chicken Soup with Coconut Milk

Prep Time: 10 Minutes

Cook Time: 30 Minutes

Servings: 6

Ingredients

- 1 Tablespoon avocado oil
- 1 Onion, diced
- 6 Cloves garlic, minced
- 2 Tablespoons Ginger paste
- 1 Tablespoon Lemongrass paste
- 2 Carrots peeled and sliced into thin coins
- 8 ounces Sliced Baby Bella mushrooms
- 6 Boneless skinless chicken thighs cut into cubes
- 2 Cups Chicken Broth
- 1 14 ounce Can coconut milk, full fat
- 3 Tablespoons Fish sauce
- 3 Tablespoons Lime juice
- 2 teaspoons Thai red curry paste
- Fresh cilantro for garnish
- Dutch Oven

Instructions

1. In a dutch oven over medium heat, add the avocado oil, onion, garlic, ginger, lemongrass and carrots.
2. Sauté until carrots begin to soften. Should take about 5-8 minutes.
3. Add in sliced mushrooms and sauté for five minutes more.

4. Add in chicken and continue to sauté until chicken is no longer pink. About 5 minutes.
5. Add in chicken broth, coconut milk, fish sauce, lime juice and red curry paste.
6. Stir and let simmer for 20 minutes uncovered.
7. Serve in bowls with cilantro for garnish.
8. Jennifer's tips
9. Ginger paste and Lemongrass paste: These 2 ingredients provide so much flavor without having to grate a ginger root, or chop a lemongrass stalk. These 2 ingredients are found in the produce section of most grocery stores.
10. Carrots: These are really not that essential to the recipe so if you want to reduce the carb count a little more, you can leave them out.

29. Keto Meatball Casserole

Prep Time: 10 Minutes

Cook Time: 35 Minutes

Servings: 6

Ingredients

- ½ Pound Ground breakfast sausage or Italian sausage
- 2 Pounds Ground beef
- ½ Cup Grated Parmesan cheese
- ⅓ cup Chopped fresh parsley
- 2 cloves Garlic, minced
- 2 Tablespoons Olive oil
- 2 Large Eggs, beaten
- 1 ½ teaspoons Kosher salt
- ½ teaspoon pepper

- 1 24 oz Jar Marinara
- 2 Cups Shredded Mozzarella Cheese

Instructions

1. Preheat your oven to 350F and spray a 9x9 casserole dish with cooking spray.
2. Combine ground beef, sausage, parmesan, parsley, olive oil, eggs, garlic, salt and pepper in a large mixing bowl. Careful not to overwork the meat.
3. Roll your mixture into 12 -13 meatballs.
4. Spray avocado oil in a large skillet and fry each meatball over medium heat until brown on all sides. Use a non stick skillet with the spray oil for even more assurance that your meatballs do not stick.
5. Place your meatballs inside a 9x9 casserole dish. Add the jar of marinara sauce around the meatballs
6. Sprinkle the shredded mozzarella cheese evenly over the top of the meatballs.
7. Bake in the oven for 20 minutes or until an internal meat thermometer reads 165F in the center of the meatballs. If you would like your cheese to get a little more brown, you can set your oven to broil for a few minutes extra.
8. Serve.
9. Jennifer's tips
10. Use Frozen Meatballs for an even quicker dish: Frozen meatballs will work in this recipe, but since frozen meatballs are generally smaller you would use more. Fill the bottom of the casserole dish with the meatballs. Note that store bought frozen meatballs are a little higher in carbs than these homemade ones.

11. Jar Marinara: The one I have linked is my favorite keto friendly marinara but you can use any brand that is your favorite. Look for one that has no sugar added. You can also make your own with my recipe for keto marinara sauce.
12. Ground Beef: I use 85/15 ground beef for this recipe
13. Pre-shredded Cheese: I always use pre-shredded cheese and this fact is reflected in the nutrition info. You can shred your own if you like.

Prep Time: 10 Minutes

Cook Time: 45 Minutes

Servings: 6

Ingredients

- 2 Tablespoons avocado oil
- kosher salt and pepper
- 1 2-4 LB Rump Roast
- 1 Cup Beef broth

For the Gravy

- 2 Tablespoons Butter
- ¼ Cup Flour or ½ teaspoon Xanthan Gum
- Beef broth for consistency

Instructions

For Instant Pot

1. Cut the roast into 4 quarters and season with salt and pepper.
2. Heat the Instant Pot using the "sauté" function on the highest setting. When the screen reads "hot" add the avocado oil.
3. Add the roast to the pot, 2 pieces at a time, and sear until a brown crust forms. Remove from the pot and set aside. Press the "cancel" button.
4. Add the beef broth to the pot and scrape any browned bits from the bottom. Add all of the roast back to the

pot, place the lid, and set the valve to "sealing." Press the "meat" function and adjust the time to 45 minutes.

5. When the cooking time is finished, let the pot naturally release the pressure for 10 minutes, then release the rest of the pressure using a quick release.
6. Remove the lid and check the roast. If it shreds easily, it is finished. If it is still tough, place the lid back on and set the timer for 15 additional minutes, followed again by a 10 minute natural release. Cooking time will depend on the size of the roast. If you are having trouble getting the lid back on, run the underside under cold water for a few seconds to cool it down.
7. After the roast is finished, remove it to a plate and set aside (leave the juices in the pot for the gravy).
8. For the gravy, set the Instant pot back on sauté and add the butter and flour or xanthan gum. Whisk thoroughly so there are no lumps and bring to a boil. If the gravy seems too thick, add beef broth a little at a time until it is your preferred thickness. Taste for seasoning and add salt an pepper if necessary.

For Crock Pot

1. Cut the roast into 4 quarters and season with salt and pepper.
2. Using a heavy bottom skillet over high heat, add the avocado oil followed by the roast. Add the roast pieces and sear on all sides until a brown crust forms. Remove from the pan and add to the Crock Pot.
3. Add the beef broth to the crock pot with the roast, place the lid, and set the Crock Pot on low for 10 hours. The roast is finished when it is easily shredded with 2 forks.
4. For the gravy, add the juices from the crock pot to a sauce pan over hi heat. Add the butter and the flour

or xanthan gum. Whisk thoroughly so there are no lumps. Bring to a boil. Add more beef broth if the gravy is too thick. Taste for seasoning and add salt and pepper if necessary.
5. Jennifer's tips
6. If you are here for low carb recipes, you will want to use the xanthan gum to thicken the gravy.

www.ingramcontent.com/pod-product-compliance
Lightning Source LLC
Chambersburg PA
CBHW071106260726
48661CB00006B/2486